Ho'oponopono:

the art of cleaning

Explore Ho'oponopono cleaning tools through coloring

Cees Maliepaard, the Hague, June 2023

"The only thing between you and Divinity is data, memory. Data is like clouds that hide the sun, but the sun is always still there. Cleaning removes the clouds... and if we could see the effects of our cleaning, we would be cleaning 24/7."
Ihaleakalae Hew Len

Ho'oponopono Cleaning tools

Introduction

Welcome to the captivating world of Ho'oponopono! This coloring book offers an opportunity for people of all ages to become acquainted with the practical cleaning tools of Ho'oponopono. The book showcases drawings of various Ho'oponopono tools mentioned in seminars by Ihaleakala Hew Len (1939-2022). As you bring these drawings to life with your colors, feel the joy and relaxation that coloring can bring and allow the wisdom of Ho'oponopono to resonate within you.

What are cleaning tools?

French philosopher Jean-Paul Sartre once described life as a journey between two points, B and D. B represents Birth, while D symbolizes Death.

Between these two points lies the letter C, which stands for Choice.

But what choice do we truly have in life?

Throughout our existence, we are faced with countless decisions, leading us to believe that our intellect or intuition guides these choices, thereby reinforcing the belief in the power of free will. However, Ho'oponopono offers a different perspective. Ho'oponopono challenges our perception of the world and teaches us that the only real choice we have is whether to live from 'memory and thinking' or 'divine inspiration'.

This choice is the only choice in life, as all other choices are ultimately illusions.

Ho'oponopono Cleaning tools

Normally, we handle problems through thinking. However, thinking is based on the memories stored in our subconscious mind. Thinking leads to chaos and confusion. Thinking looks outside of ourselves. For example, if we have trouble with our spouse, thinking leads us to believe that the cause lies with the spouse. But in Ho'oponopono, we say, *"there is no out there."* The cause is always within us.

In Ho'oponopono, cleaning tools serve as the key to becoming free from our memories and our memory-based thinking. Cleaning works within ourselves, where the memories reside that are the cause of our problems and diseases. Cleaning is about 'allowing' the resolution of the problem and bringing peace to the situation. Cleaning is about creating a peaceful relationship with Divinity/Love/God/Light/Creator (whatever words suit you) and receiving divine guidance on how to act. Cleaning fosters positive changes in our lives.

However, we must acknowledge that we have only one choice, and we must take 100% responsibility: life is an inside job, and memories never fade away unless we actively release them using these cleaning tools.

In short, we can choose how to live and how to act. We can act based on:
a. the battery power of memories and thinking or
b. the full power of the Divine. If you choose the latter, you can use these cleaning tools because they are the key to erasing memories in our subconscious mind, allowing us to receive divine guidance and create positive change in our lives.

Ho'oponopono Cleaning tools

Why are there so many cleaning tools?
When asked about the abundance of cleaning tools, Hew Len drew a parallel to a wardrobe. Look in your wardrobe, he said. Each item of clothing is intended for a special occasion. You don't wear garden clothes to a wedding. It is the same with the cleaning tools: you can use them according to your needs. Choose a specific cleaning tool to work with, or combine them based on your needs.

Which cleaning tools are we discussing?
In this coloring book, we explore 11 cleaning tools:

1. I love you
2. Thank you
3. Please forgive me
4. I'm sorry
5. Light switch
6. Blue solar water
7. Ice Blue
8. Dew Drop and eraser
9. HA-breathing
10. Strawberries
11. Glas of water tool

These cleaning tools are not explicitly refer to a particular situation, but they serve as activation words to release worries, beliefs, judgments, and anything that distracts us from the present moment. They are a means of opening ourselves to what is right and perfect, allowing it to unfold naturally.

Ho'oponopono Cleaning tools

The Ho'oponopono activation words or phrases serve as a way to give permission for the memories replaying in our subconscious mind to be erased by Divinity.

Keep in mind that Ho'oponopono cleaning is not limited to a specific situation, as we can never be certain which memory is playing out or what needs to unfold. Even physical ailments are memories that arise to provide us with an opportunity to release and cleanse.

Whether you are a child, a teenager, a parent, or a grandparent, this coloring book invites you in an active way to discover the beauty and power of Ho'oponopono cleaning tools.

So, dear readers don't hesitate, grab your coloring tools, young and old alike. As you breathe life into these illustrations with colors, immerse yourself in the joy of coloring and allow the wisdom of Ho'oponopono to resonate within you.

Enjoy your coloring adventure and embrace Ho'oponopono!

Cleaning tool 1-4: the 4 sentences

The most famous and widely used cleaning tools are 'I'm sorry,' 'Thank you,' 'Please forgive me,' and 'I love you.' These powerful tools were described in Joe Vitale's popular book, 'Zero Limits.'

Utilizing these simple tools is easy: repeat the sentences either silently or aloud. It doesn't matter which you choose; go with what suits you best. Say the sentences without any attachment or expectations; be open and flexible. You never know what may develop as a result of uttering these sentences.

By saying these phrases we come to the realization that we don't know anything. By saying these sentences, we allow the part of us that knows better, holds solutions to all our problems, to inspire us and bring us what is perfect and right at the ideal moment. When you are coloring say softly or think: 'I'm sorry,' 'Thank you,' 'Please forgive me' and 'I love you'.

I love you

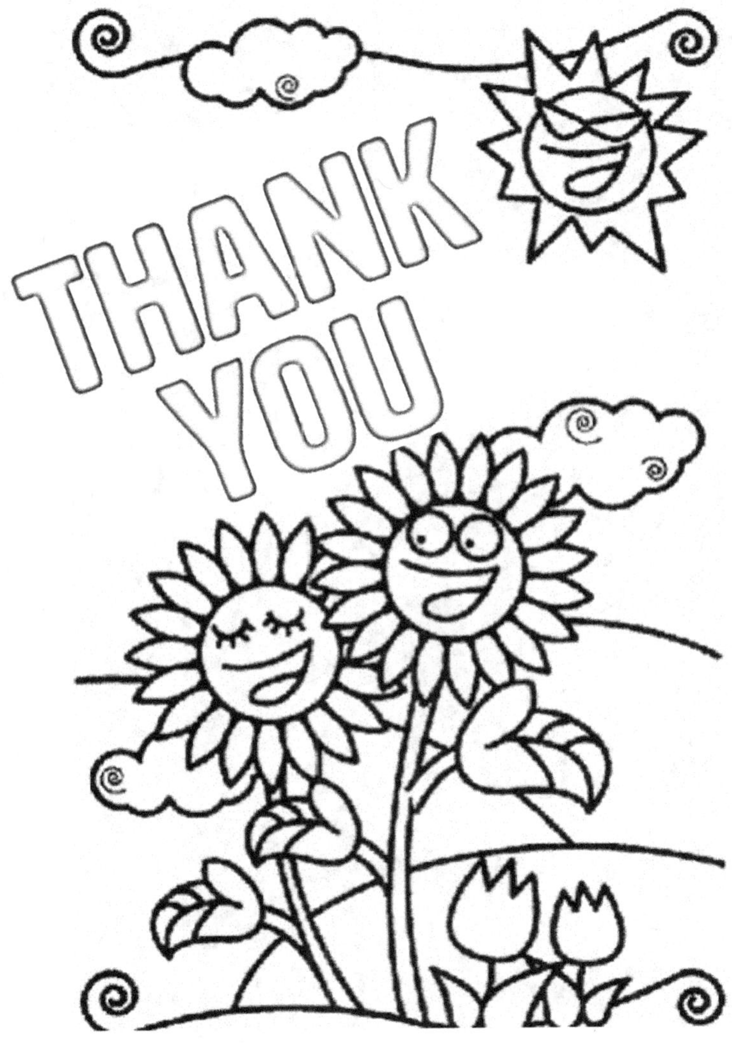
THANK YOU

Ho'oponopono Cleaning tools

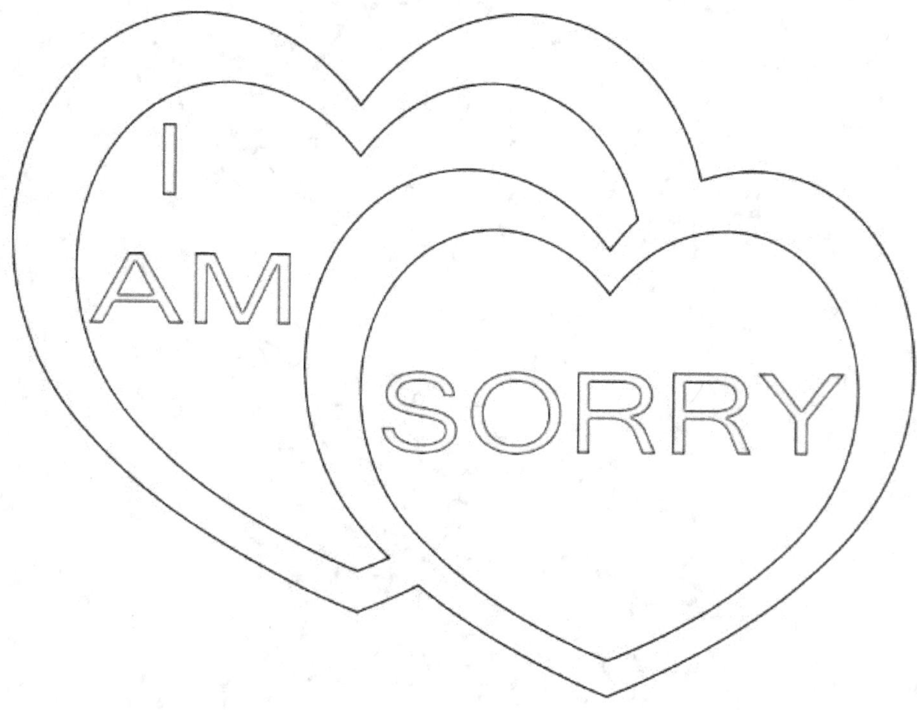

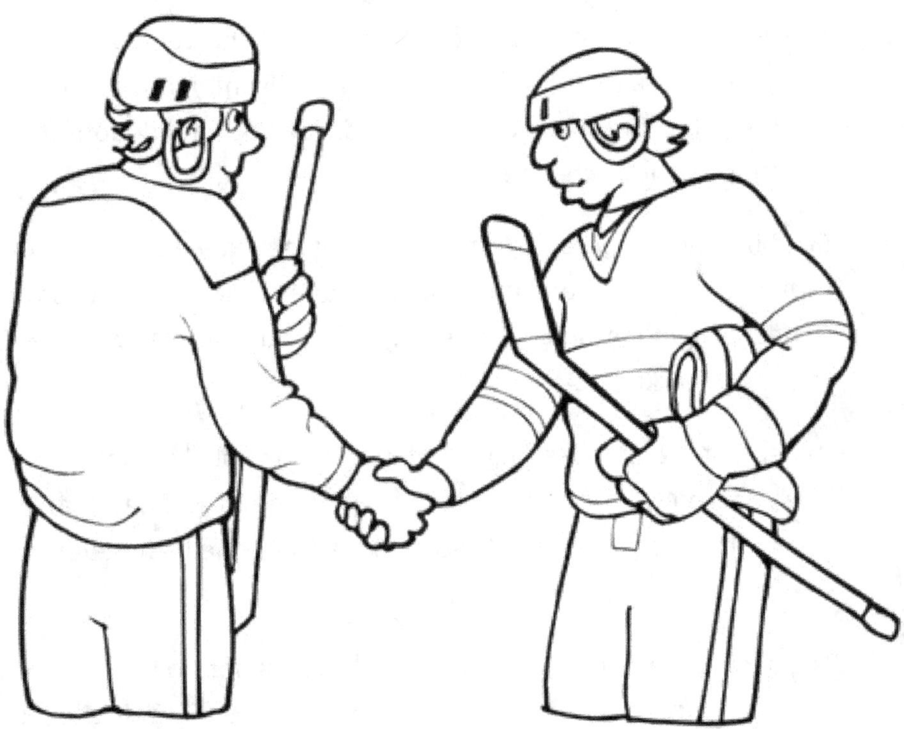
Please forgive me

Cleaning tool 5: the Light Switch

The Light Switch serves as a powerful symbol of your ability to illuminate awareness and bring clarity to challenging situations or negative thoughts. Visualize the act of mentally turning on the Light Switch and affirm, *"I activate the Light Switch for myself, my family, relatives, and ancestors."* This tool has no limits on its usage. It is a heartfelt plea to Divinity, requesting the clearance of toxic thoughts that divide your mind, both for yourself and your lineage.

Even if only one person in the room engages this tool, the light radiates for all. It represents the memories that have blocked Divinity's light within us. By neglecting to turn on the light, we remain in darkness.

Repeating the phrases "light switch," "thank you," or "I love you" internally is equivalent to activating the light. Regardless of who initiates it, the light radiates for everyone. Whatever is erased within you is erased for all.

To practice Ho'oponopono is to grant permission to Divinity to erase negativity within you and fill your life with light. It guides you towards happiness and inner peace, regardless of the external circumstances surrounding you.

Ho'oponopono Cleaning tools

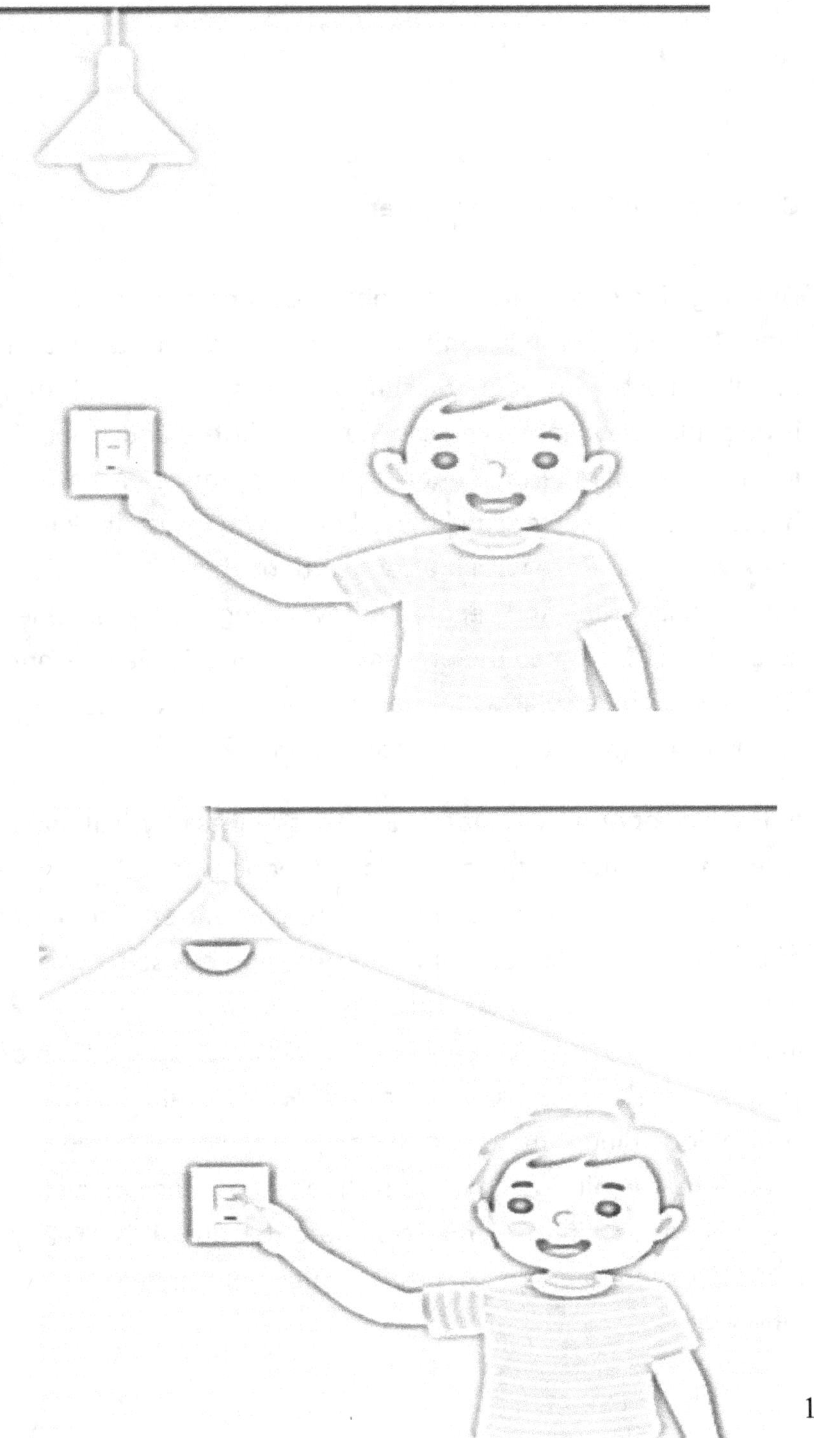

Cleaning tool 6: Blue Solar water

Drinking blue solar water is a problem-solving process. Get a blue glass bottle with a nonmetallic cover and pour tap water into it. Place the bottle in the sun for at least one hour. If there is no sunlight available, you can place the bottle under an incandescent lamp (not a fluorescent lamp) for at least an hour. Blue solar water can be used in several ways: drink it, cook with it, or rinse with it after a bath or shower. Additionally, fruits and vegetables love being washed in blue solar water! Similar to the processes of saying 'I love you' and 'Thank you,' blue solar water helps eliminate memories that replay problems in the subconscious mind.

In Ho'oponopono, imagination is just as real as physical reality. One of the central themes in Ho'oponopono is the idea that *"there is no out there"*. But what about blue water? Isn't it part of the outside world? Certainly, because you can see it with your eyes. However, what you cannot see -and that's the key in Ho'oponopono - is that the solar water holds a reflection of your inner self. When you create solar water, it aligns with your unique blueprint and not with someone else's blueprint. Therefore, the blue solar water is different for each individual. You will not obtain the same solar water because it is already meant or preordained to perfectly match your unique blueprint.

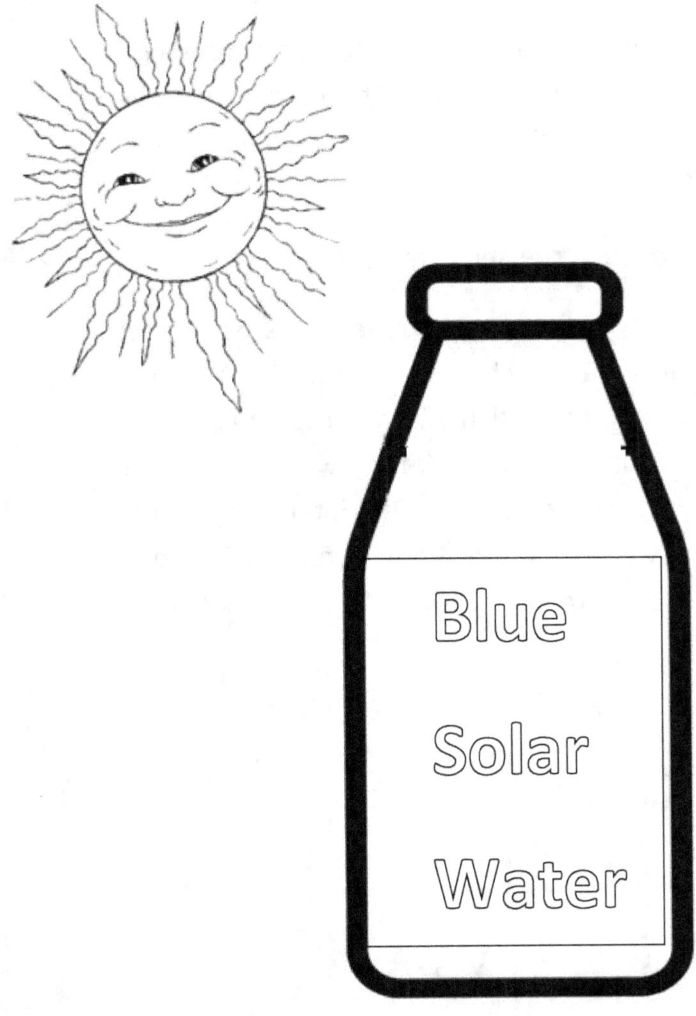

Blue
Solar
Water

Cleaning tool 7: Ice blue

"Ice Blue" is effective in alleviating any pain and suffering. Simply think "ice blue" when you have burns, cuts, bruises, or any kind of discomfort. Utilize it while cutting plants and grass to help numb their pain.

When walking, touch a tree and utter "Ice Blue."

Feel free to use it as frequently as needed to assist yourself, others, or anything that may be experiencing distress. This approach aligns with the fundamental principle of Ho'oponopono—taking 100% responsibility for what unfolds in our daily lives, moment by moment. The intention is to repeat this phrase without expectations, even if the annoyance persists. Just continue to let go.

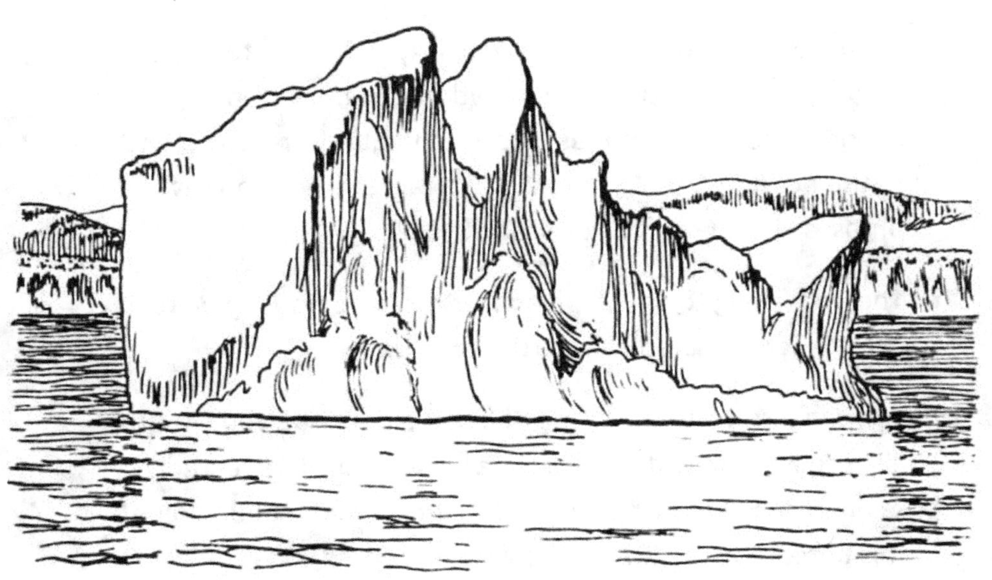

Ho'oponopono Cleaning tools

Cleaning tool 8: dewdrop and eraser

You can utilize the Ho'oponopono cleaning tools called "Dewdrop" and "Eraser" when you experience fear, threat, sadness, or anger. Use it moment to moment.

Grab a pencil with an eraser and lightly tap on an item such as a book, computer, picture, or anything else. This tapping action erases all memories across generations, reaching back to the point of their creation. While tapping, you can say phrases like "Dewdrop" or "Thank you."

These cleaning tools can be applied to any emotion you're experiencing related to a particular situation.

You can also write the name of a person or issue you wish to cleanse and tap with the eraser end of a pencil, repeatedly saying "Dewdrop" whenever it bothers you. Continue doing this until there are no more issues associated with it.

Ho'oponopono Cleaning tools

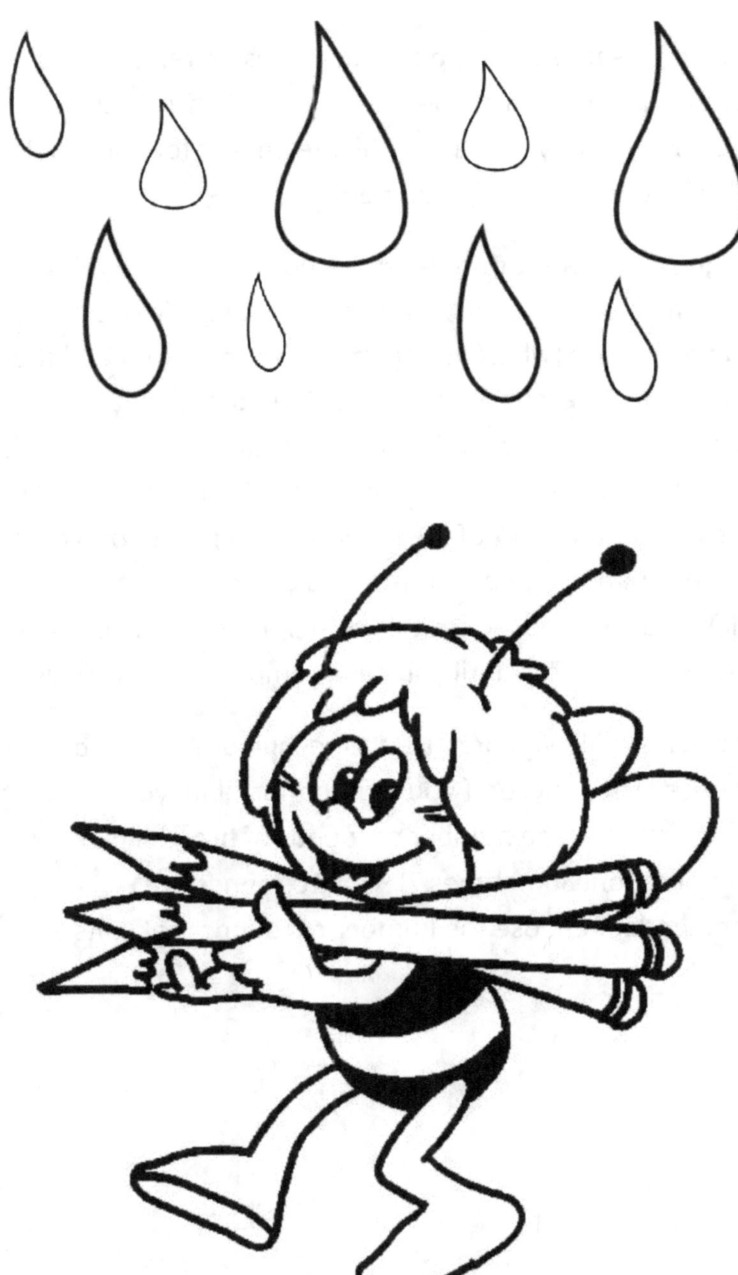

Ho'oponopono Cleaning tools

Cleaning tool 9: HA-breathing

The act of breathing in Ho'oponopono has no relation to a physical process for example, the increased absorption of oxygen by the body. It is a mental one, meant for your soul. It involves the transmutation of memories.

To begin, assume a comfortable seated position and bring your thumb and index finger together, symbolizing the oneness of God and yourself (where the thumb represents God and the index finger represents you). Take a deep breath in through your nose, counting to 10 (feel free to count at your own pace, whether it's fast or slow). Hold your breath for a count of 10, then exhale for a count of 10, followed by a pause for a count of 10. Each complete cycle is considered one round. Begin the inhalation again, and repeat this cycle for a total of 10 rounds. Continue the process until you have completed ten rounds.

How often should you practice this technique? Aim to do it at least once every day, or if you feel comfortable, you can do it more frequently. The number of rounds of breathing depends on the situation. Sometimes 7, 9, or 10 rounds are recommended. Choose the number of rounds that suits you.

1 2 3 4

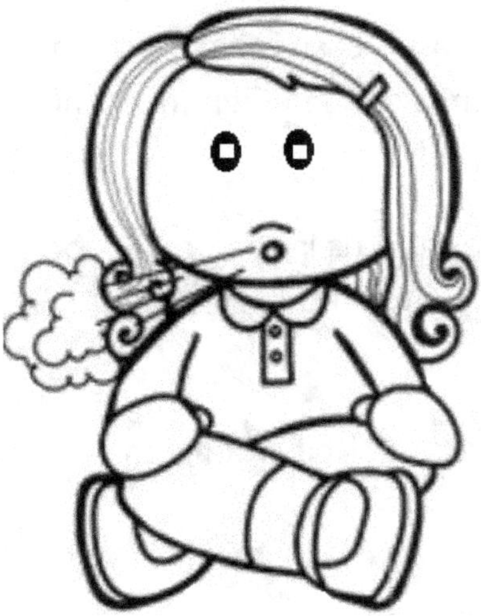

5 6

7

Ho'oponopono Cleaning tools

Cleaning tool 10: Strawberries

Include strawberries in your diet, whether fresh, dried, in jam, or in ice cream, as they have the power to heal the heart and alleviate depression. Consume fresh or frozen strawberries, or strawberry jam. This practice helps release memories and thoughts that manifest as concerns about weight (not only physical but also mental).

The consumption of strawberries aids us in the process of cleaning. It supports our journey towards balance and freedom.

Additionally, this healing process can also be done on a mental level: think e.g. strawberrie.

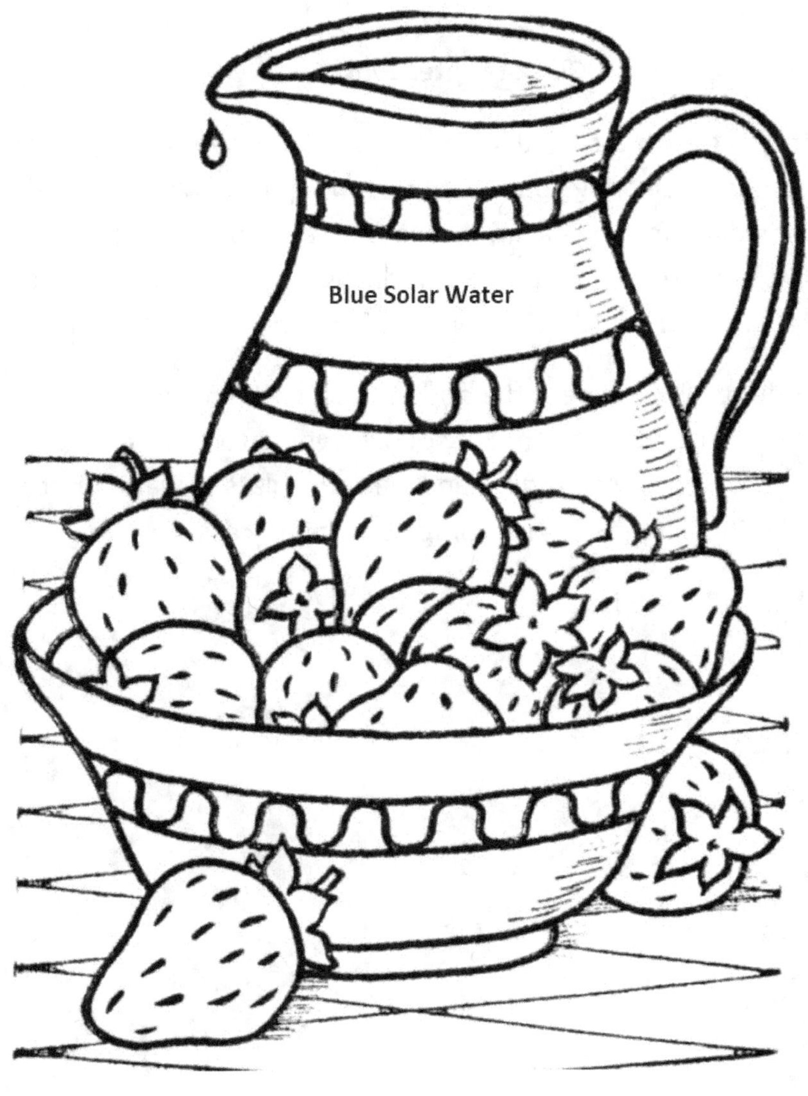
Blue Solar Water

Cleaning tool 11: Glas of Water tool.

Place a clear glass filled at least ¾ full with water in your home to assist in clearing your memories when they are not in your immediate focus. Change the water in the glass at least twice a day, or more frequently if desired. The glass acts as a vessel to transmute the negative energies of memories and thoughts.

Additionally, you have the option to write the name of a person or a situation that is troubling you on a piece of paper (e.g. *"how to pay this bill"*) and place the glass of water on top of it. This simple practice completes the process.

That's all there is to it.

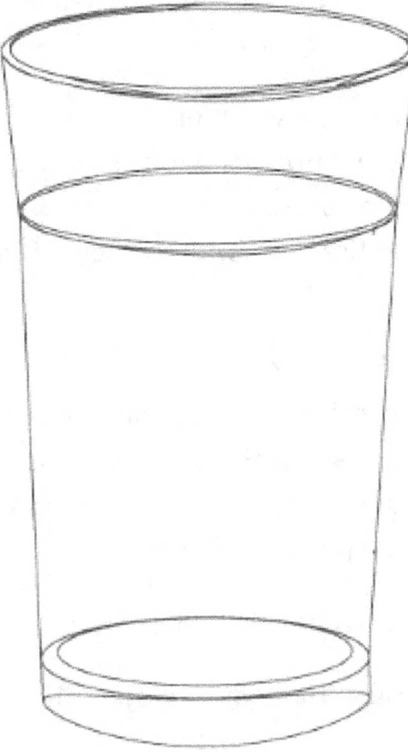

Ho'oponopono Cleaning tools

Closing remarks

Regardless of your age, this coloring book is a gateway to get acquainted with the Ho'oponopon cleaning tools. By coloring, the tools become more personal and hopefully it stimulates you to apply them practically.

Every color holds its own vibration. Let the synergy of colors, the cleaning tools and Ho'oponopono's wisdom guide you on your path of freeing yourself. Remember: memories never retire unless you retire them with the help of these cleaning tools!

May this coloring book also serve as an inspiration to delve deeper into the teachings of Ho'oponopono. Explore my other easy-to-read ebooks about Ho'oponopono, so that you can gain a better understanding of what Ho'oponopono can mean for you. Ho'oponopono is truly profound.

You can find these ebooks on amazon.com:

Ho'oponopono: the pitfall!: a short story that unlocks the secret of life
This ebook tells the story of a family facing challenges, where Grandpa shows them the way to solve their problems using Ho'oponopono. And guess what? It works! It is written in an accessible manner suitable for readers of all ages.

Ho'oponopono Cleaning tools

Ho'oponopono: beyond thinking

This short introduction to Ho'oponopono describes its principles, provides practical examples, and much more. According to a reader: *"A very helpful guide and reminder"*.

Ho'oponopono: dowsing at zero

What is dowsing? In short: dowsing is a way to get answers on questions we cannot get with our senses/rational mind. The use of dowsing is infinite. It is about finding lost objects, it's about the best place to go on holiday, it's about vitamin deficiency, it's about the volt of a battery, it's about questions like: "is a painting from Banksy or not…".
A must-read for those who comprehend that nature holds more significance than our intellect.

Ho'oponopono: Suzanne by Leonard Cohen Explained

Do you believe that the Bible or the Bhagavad Gītā are the sole books that provide insights into life? Even in modern times, we come across signs, but we must be observant to notice them. Read this ebook about the beautiful song "Suzanne" by Leonard Cohen and be amazed.

Ho'oponopono: a new take on Queen's Bohemian Rhapsody

A review tells all: *"Your mind is about to be blown! I'm in awe of the authors insight into Bohemian Rhapsody from the Ho'oponopono perspective! If you want to have a huge aha moment in a very short period of time, give yourself the gift of the next 15-20 minutes to read this little gem! You will be so glad you did!!! "*

Ho'oponopono: beyond medical knowledge
There is much more to healing than the limited medical knowledge of today. While our intellect may not fully comprehend it, this ebook offers a different perspective that explores the depths of healing. A reader wrote: *"This book is a must read. Very simple and to the point clearly describing how to clean our subconscious and hence heal ourselves."*

Let this coloring book serve as a reminder that regardless of our age, we all possess the ability to learn, grow, and cultivate inner peace, which can in turn radiate through our community, society, nation, and the Universe!